Stephen Pollard is Chief Leader Writer of *The Express* and co-author of
Ready for Treatment, published by the Social Market Foundation in 1997.
Katharine Raymond is Director of the Social Market Foundation.

A Question of Choice

Public Priorities for Health Care

STEPHEN POLLARD and
KATHARINE RAYMOND

The Social Market Foundation
September 1999

First published in English by The Social Market Foundation, 1999
in association with Profile Books Ltd

The Social Market Foundation
11 Tufton Street
London SW1P 3QB

Profile Books Ltd
58A Hatton Garden
London ECIN 8LX

Typeset in Bembo by MacGuru
macguru@pavilion.co.uk

Printed in Great Britain by Hobbs the Printers

A CIP catalogue record for this book is available from the British Library.

Paper No. 43

ISBN 1 874097 59 3

Contents

The authors are grateful to
Nick Sparrow at ICM and to Pfizer Inc.
for their support.

Introduction

Britain's National Health Service is still the most revered of all British institutions – the monarchy included – thanks to its unique ability to deliver health care free at point of use, universally.

The NHS, however, is far from perfect. Demand for any good provided at zero cost is bound to be infinite, and policy makers have long considered how the existing model could best be adapted to cope with new, modern-day pressures.

Two years ago the Social Market Foundation (SMF) conducted the most extensive opinion poll ever on what the public expected from the NHS in the future. The basic public assumption was that, in ten years time, the NHS would charge for certain treatments and services. It would continue to provide a core service, but beyond that patients would have to make their own, private, arrangements.

A Question of Choice is the result of a new ICM survey which aimed to dig deeper behind the original findings of 1997. The results show clearly that the public is far more realistic about the likely developments in health care than governments and policy analysts give them credit for.

The British public is, it seems, becoming far more aware of rationing – not only in terms of the length of time spent waiting for treatment, but also in terms of the lack in choice in treatment.

Despite there being more information available about diseases and their treatments than ever before, the range of treatments is becoming steadily more restricted. The new National Institute for Clinical Excellence is a case in point. There is an emerging conflict between the desire for a greater range of choice and problems arising from the rationing made inevitable by the NHS' funding mechanism. Something, sooner or later, will have to give.

The public clearly understands that none of these issues can be addressed without dealing with funding. It wants extra money to be spent on reducing waiting lists *and* on having available more of the latest and most effective treatments. But voters, it seems, do not trust politicians to target any extra resources properly, and many claim that they would prefer a hypothecated health tax.

Attitudes towards funding change when people consider how they personally might have to contribute. Asked where their own money should go, they say on better consultations with their doctors, on a wider choice of treatments and on ensuring prompt, reliable appointments. So-called 'public money', on the other hand, should be spent on smarter surgeries and better pay for doctors and nurses.

What emerges most clearly is that, despite the attachment to a NHS and health care funded exclusively out of taxation, voters consider such a model to be in its death throes. They do not welcome the 'end' of the NHS as we know it today, but they do expect it.

That means that they also expect to have to make some kind of regular payment for their future health care, either within the NHS (such as for GP visits) or via a 'top up' mechanism, perhaps involving private insurance. None of this looks or sounds like practical politics today. But the British public is often ahead of its politicians, and this survey confirms that they appreciate and understand the irreversible logic at the heart of the NHS' problems. Tax revenue can only be stretched so far, and with demand and costs on a constant and unavoidable upward path, the extra funding needed to make up the difference will have to be found elsewhere.

Stephen Pollard and Katharine Raymond, *September 1999*

Executive Summary

In 1997 the Social Market Foundation published *Ready for Treatment*, the largest survey ever conducted of the public's expectations about the future of the National Health Service. In that study the authors described the fundamental issue for policy makers as the 'expectations gap'. In other words, that the public wants the NHS to offer everything to everyone, and to offer it free of charge. But while more than 65 per cent of those questioned think that NHS treatments should always be free at the point of use, very few actually believe that they will be in the future.

Crucially, only 13 per cent expect existing NHS services to be free of charge in a decade. Well over two thirds think that the NHS will provide fewer services, and that those no longer offered will be available only privately; and 62 per cent expect some form of additional charges in the NHS within the next decade.

Despite their general satisfaction with the standard of service, voters had a sense that the NHS had drifted away from their priorities due to the internal market, and that its focus no longer adequately reflected public wishes. Labour had campaigned in opposition almost exclusively on one health-care-related issue – the length of waiting lists. It pledged that a Labour government would see a dramatic reduction in waiting times. After some initial delay, the energy and the funds directed towards that end are beginning to have an effect, although this may prove to be short-term, given the continuing 'expectations gap'.

Since the 1997 survey, the government has taken action by instituting the National Institute of Clinical Excellence (NICE) prescribing guidelines, and by recommending the 'doctor-prompting' PRODIGY prescribing tools, both of which have the capability of limiting choice and restricting access to new medicines, thereby increasing the feasibility of greater rationing of new therapies.

Building from the previous study, *A Question of Choice* explores in more detail the public's expectations and concerns about the future of the NHS. The aim of the study was to evaluate the public's views and major concerns about the NHS, their level and sources of knowledge, and their preferred options for addressing those concerns.

The key themes which emerge from the survey are three-fold:

- Across the board the public has a sense that it is being denied access through rationing. Rationing is perceived in two ways; not only by queues for treatment, but also in the limitation of choice among therapies – notably for new medicines.
- The public has a distinct preference that funds be targeted or dedicated towards addressing their major concerns – especially those related to rationing. Without such action, 67 per cent of the public expects that the situation will stay the same or worsen.
- There is a large information disparity between those who are frequent users of the NHS and those who are

not. The public does expect to have wider sources of information and to be better informed in the future. This raises the prospect that unless greater choice is available to patients, dissatisfaction will increase.

The following is a synopsis of the survey's findings. It addresses the key issues of how much the public knows about the NHS; how frequently they use it; and the extent to which they participate in decisions. It also examines their major concerns, priorities and preferred options for change.

Note: numbers in the tables may not add up to exactly 100% due to rounding.

Commentary on the
Public Opinion Survey

How much do people use NHS services?

There are two aspects to this question: what proportion of people use the services, and how much use do those people make of the services?

	Percentage having used the service in the last year
NHS doctor	66
Accident and Emergency department	15
Other hospital	22
NHS dentist	40

The most widely used NHS service is the local GP. The first point of contact for most patients with the NHS is at the GP's surgery. Two thirds (66 per cent) of people have visited their GP at least once in the past year.

Age is a useful indicator of usage rates of the NHS.

	18–24 (per cent)	25–44 (per cent)	45–64 (per cent)	65+ (per cent)
NHS doctor	58	65	64	74
A&E	18	22	11	9
Other hospital	11	21	20	29
NHS dentist	43	47	38	26

Dental and casualty treatment tend to decline with age, but older people make much more use of GPs and hospitals. There is also a difference with regard to sex, with women making more use of the range of services than men do. This is particularly the case with the GP service (73 per cent of women, 57 per cent of men) and hospital (26 per cent and 17 per cent).

There are several possible causes of the greater exposure of women to the NHS. Longer female life expectancy means that most people aged over 75, the heaviest consumers of NHS services, are women. For some younger women, pregnancy involves prolonged contact with the health service, and there are periodic women's health checks which have no male equivalent. Working patterns also affect the use of doctors, with 57 per cent of people working full time doing so and 72 per cent of the rest of the population. This is, of course, correlated with the age and sex factors already mentioned.

Use of other NHS facilities tends to be associated with seeing a GP; over 90 per cent of those using hospitals either for A&E or non-emergency care in the last year have also seen their doctor. It is a safe assumption that a person who has used hospital services has either been seen first by a GP or will be seen later for follow-up examinations and treatment.

Satisfaction with NHS services

Most people who use the NHS are happy with the standard of service they receive.

	Very satisfied (per cent)	Very unsatisfied (per cent)	Mean score
NHS doctor	47	2	1.33
A&E	35	6	0.93
Other hospital	43	3	1.16
NHS dentist	44	1	1.33

The mean score is calculated by giving answers a value from +2 for 'very satisfied' to −2 for 'very unsatisfied' and then taking an average. The public are clearly impressed with NHS doctors and dentists, although a little more critical of the quality of accident and emergency units: even in that case the proportion satisfied exceeds the proportion dissatisfied (78 per cent and 18 per cent).

The high level of satisfaction is remarkably constant across age, sex and class divides, although the wealthier patients (higher-rate taxpayers) were slightly more critical of NHS doctors (satisfaction mean score 1.00, compared to 1.36 for basic rate taxpayers).

The public overwhelmingly feel that staff commitment (97 per cent) and increased funding (96 per cent) are important factors in determining the quality of treatment. Support for this view varied little between supporters of the different political parties. Three quarters consider both factors very important, and they are clearly of a different order of importance from other factors.

Patients also feel that Community Health Councils (78 per cent) and the Patient's Charter (79 per cent) are important in keeping up standards, with only 12 per cent and 9 per cent respectively considering them not very or not at all important. Just over three quarters (76 per cent) think that an attitude of customer service, not just regarding people as patients, is very or quite important, although 19 per cent disagree.

There is less consensus on the importance of modern buildings, 70 per cent agreeing (although not very strongly) and 28 per cent not rating this as important.

Patients as consumers

There is an almost even divide among the public between those who think that doctors fully discuss their illness and treatment and those who do not. However, it is worth noting that there is a cluster of particularly heavy users of health services: 24 per cent of those visiting a GP did so six or more times in the preceding year (18 per cent of the whole population) and 36 per cent of these heavy users also made two or more visits to hospital over the same period, compared to 15 per cent among all GP patients.

Not surprisingly, the more frequently a patient uses the health service, the more fully he or she tends to feel that doctors engage in full discussion. Six out of ten (60 per cent) of those with repeated hospital visits felt their GP discussed matters fully with them. Age also made a difference, with 55 per cent of those aged over 65 thinking that their doctor discussed matters fully.

Generally, though, discussions with doctors are perceived to be good, as nearly half of all respondents claim their doctor fully discussed what was wrong with them and nearly a third that their problem was discussed briefly.

	All respondents (per cent)	Men (per cent)	Women (per cent)
Fully	45	42	48
Briefly	30	27	32
Hardly at all	11	11	11
Never	2	2	2
Not applicable	12	18	7

In contrast to the discussion of their illness, however, the majority did not consider they were given a choice of treatment. Most patients surveyed did not play an active part in the prescribing decisions of their doctor.

Only a small minority appear to participate in an active, 'consumer' sense in clinical decisions that affect them; the proportion rises a little among the heaviest users of health services (14 per cent of those attending 6 or more times a year say they are always given a choice). Even among people who have at some stage been offered a choice, less than half (47 per cent) of the patients feel that it is a fully informed choice in which the doctor has explained all the options. Considerably less than half (42 per cent) say that the choice is briefly explained, and 9 per cent hardly at all.

When given a choice, options were	(per cent)
Fully explained	47
Briefly explained	42
Hardly explained at all	9
DK	2

The passive nature of the prescribing transaction is also shown when respondents were asked to speculate on how their doctor would respond if they asked for a specific course of treatment.

	(per cent)
Prescribe what they were going to prescribe me anyway	38
Prescribe it to me unless there were good clinical grounds not to do so	35
Offer me something else but explain the reasons why	25
DK	2

These proportions did not vary much by age, sex or class, although people who have frequent dealings with the health service tended to be more confident that their judgement would be followed.

Since the answers in the above table are not mutually exclusive, the data can be interpreted in two ways: either that only 35 per cent would expect their choice to be respected, unless there were good clinical grounds not to do so, or that a total of 63 per cent would not expect to have an effect on their GP's decision to prescribe a particular drug.

Most people see prescription medicine as a professional decision taken by the doctor and not a 'consumer choice' in the commonly understood sense of the term. When the decision has been made, most patients feel that the doctor has informed them about relevant issues.

When you are given a prescription by your doctor, is any of the following explained to you?	percentage responding 'Yes'
The name of the drug	57
Its ingredients	26
What it is supposed to do	76
If it has any potential side-effects	68

At the extreme, 14 per cent are told absolutely nothing, while 23 per cent are told all four facts about their medicine. It is surprising to note that 26 per cent claim to be told about the composition of the drug; it would seem unlikely that a quarter of the population have the pharmacological knowledge to make sense of such information. All these facts are usually found in information leaflets included with packets of medication and can also be ascertained from pharmacists. The survey did not show how many patients were offered different treatments or a choice of medicines.

The response to charging

In the 1997 survey reported in *Ready for Treatment*, the public expected that during the next ten years they would have to pay charges for some NHS services which are currently provided free at the point of delivery. Indeed, 63 per cent thought that it was likely, although 48 per cent were strongly opposed.

It is striking that, shortly after the election of the Labour government in May 1997, a majority thought that the government would be introducing charges against their personal wishes in the foreseeable future. An overwhelming majority (91 per cent) felt that the NHS should provide GP services free, but only 53 per cent thought that it would be doing so in 2007.

This survey explored the more detailed attitudes to what else patients would expect from doctor's appointments if a £10 charge were to be introduced. Most respondents thought that they would be entitled to a higher standard of service if they were obliged to pay for it. When they were asked, if a £10 charge were introduced for a GP visit, what would be expected in return, the far highest-ranking expectations relate to easier and more timely access to the GP and more information about their illness and choice of treatment.

Patients would expect a less overloaded service with realistic appointment times and a shorter gap between realising the need to be seen by the doctor and the appointment time.

Associated with this demand is more communication between doctor and patient, with more information being given about the illness and how it will be treated and longer appointment times to allow patient and doctor to explore the issues.

	Percentage expecting
To get a fast/immediate appointment	91
To be seen at the appointed time	89
More information about illness and treatment	85
To be given more time by the doctor	81
To be visited by the doctor	71
More operations conducted at GP's surgery	51
Better waiting rooms	49
To be seen by the doctor even if a nurse could attend	43

A large proportion of respondents wanted an unprecedented level of service, including 43 per cent who said they would insist on being seen by a doctor rather than a nurse even when the latter were qualified. If a question in the survey had asked if people would expect free tea and biscuits while waiting for their appointment it would surely have attracted considerable support!

A charge might unleash a more demanding and, perhaps, even unreasonable approach by consumers who think they are entitled to a perfect service because they have paid a direct charge for it. This conflicts with the way respondents say they would like the revenue raised by the hypothetical charge to be spent.

The results suggest that there is some ambiguity about who sets 'national' priorities for the NHS. Whilst respondents generally favoured paying into an overall fund, they also wanted to know what the additional funds would pay for. Only 21 per cent of respondents wanted to direct the extra money to fund additional time for patient consultations with doctors; the rest see it as a contribution to a general pool of NHS funding.

Despite this, the latter would nevertheless like it to be allocated according to their own priorities. Whether these priorities should be decided via some form of hypothecated tax or via patient consultation remains unclear.

	Percentage choosing
To allow doctors to spend more time on patients	21
To cut hospital waiting lists	44
To prevent some treatments from being rationed	22
To pay doctors and nurses more	9
To improve facilities for patients in hospital	8
DK	1

Of course, charging would not only improve the service by increasing the overall funding base of the NHS but could also improve the GP service by reducing the often frivolous demand for appointments. Most people (85 per cent against

14 per cent) would not consult their doctor about minor illnesses such as a heavy cold or flu if there were a £10 charge, and by a similar margin thought that people they knew would not do so either.

Going to the pharmacy and buying over-the-counter drugs would become more cost-effective and most doctors would advise people to do this anyway. The 1997 survey found that 64 per cent admitted that they sometimes saw their doctor without particularly good reason, so an estimate of the proportion of people whose behaviour would be affected in this way by a charge would be around 40 to 50 per cent.

GPs might also lose some of their current role as gate-keepers to the hospital system. If the patient expected that a doctor would refer him or her to hospital, 65 per cent would go directly to the hospital if allowed to do so, and only 34 per cent would consult the doctor first. While freeing up the GP service, this might impose an extra burden on hospitals though it seems logical that a gatekeeper requirement would be imposed.

Public knowledge about personal health
More health knowledge is associated with being female, middle-aged and affluent – and of course with being a repeat customer of health services. When asked whether their knowledge about health had changed over the last five years, only a tiny proportion admitted that it had got worse; the rest were evenly divided (49 per cent improved, 47 per cent no change).

Percentage considering themselves…	All	Men	Women	18–24	Higher rate tax	Hospital 2+ times
Very or reasonably knowledgeable	50	47	52	39	63	58
Having some or little knowledge	44	45	43	51	34	40
Having no knowledge	6	8	5	10	3	2

The strongest effect on knowledge seems to have been from coming into contact with hospital, both accident and emergency and other services. Frequency of seeing a GP does not seem a great influence in people's self-assessed state of health knowledge.

When asked where they get information about personal health, people name a variety of sources. The mainstream media are the most important source of knowledge. GPs are the second most important source overall, and the most important source among people who have visited them more than once in the last year. Considering the lack of communication nearly half of patients report when they see their doctors, it is clear that when doctors do comment and explain people take it very seriously.

New systems such as advice lines, kiosks and the Internet are as yet of relatively little significance and presumably still used alongside traditional ways of obtaining information. Asked to look to the future, only a minority anticipated using them more over the next ten years. The source which the largest number of people (31 per cent) expected to use more was their GP.

According to the survey, the current pattern of passive consumption of advice from the media and doctors is considered likely to continue. While the 'parent–child' relationship in health care is a general trend it does, however, seem likely, given evidence from other countries where new technologies are more widespread, that patients will become more informed and begin taking a more active role in health care decisions as these sources of information continue to develop.

	Percentage obtaining information
MEDIA	
Magazines and newspapers	45
TV and radio	41
FORMAL SOURCES	
Your GP	44
Pharmacist	22
Official literature and advertising	15
Telephone advice lines	2
Information kiosks	1
INFORMAL SOURCES	
Friends and relatives	34
Friends and relatives working in health	13
Reference books and CD ROMs	13
Internet	3
No information or sources	15

Rationing

Most of the public believe that rationing operates informally within the NHS already, either via treatments and/or services not being freely available to everybody or else by means of waiting lists. The following table, however, demonstrates clearly the public's confusion over what is, in reality, rationed and what is not.

Percentage believing	Rationed	Not rationed	Don't know
Cancer screening	41	55	4
Dentistry	49	46	5
Heart operations for the elderly	62	34	4
The latest and most effective drugs and treatments	67	29	4
Infertility treatment	76	19	5
Tattoo removals	79	16	5
Cosmetic surgery	80	16	4

Dentistry has been rationed by price since 1951, and since the late 1980s NHS dental treatment has become scarce in some parts of the country.

It is also curious that as many as 41 per cent think cancer screening is rationed, given that it is not rationed at all, although some treatments are, and that extensive coverage of clinically determined risk groups is the point of such programmes.

The finding that 67 per cent of people think the latest drugs are rationed is significant, particularly as the survey was conducted before the introduction of the NICE and PRODIGY guidelines. A common concern was that new treatments would be rationed on the grounds of cost, and patients would be prescribed older and less effective treatments instead.

Asked whether they were personally concerned by this prospect, as many as 71 per cent said that they were concerned or very concerned and only 7 per cent professed not to be at all concerned by rationing.

Expressions of concern about rationing	All respondents (per cent)	Male (per cent)	Female (per cent)
Very concerned	33	31	36
Concerned	38	38	37
A little concerned	21	21	21
Not at all concerned	7	10	5
DK	1	0	1

Looking to the future, 67 per cent of people expect NHS rationing to stay the same or increase over the next ten years, as new drugs and treatments are developed as a result of scientific research. As many as 69 per cent also think that waiting lists will remain the same or worsen.

Interestingly, about a third of those surveyed (33 per cent) think that scientific advances might help the productivity of the NHS, although it is probable that new medical advances will actually increase pressure on the NHS either by increasing life expectancy or by increasing demand for new and better treatments.

Percentage expecting in ten years:	Problem of NHS rationing	Length of waiting lists
Better	33	31
Stay the same	27	26
Worse	40	43

Paying for better treatments

Asked whether they would be willing to pay more for treatments, either through charging or income tax increases, the public was split. Support depended both on *which* treatments they were asked to pay for and *how* they were asked to pay for them. As many as 71 per cent were willing to pay more for the latest and most effective drugs and treatments, while only 6 per cent were willing to pay extra for 'non-core' treatments like tattoo removal.

Willingness to pay is, not unsurprisingly, correlated with ability to pay: 59 per cent of the 25–44 age group and 66 per cent of higher-rate taxpayers are willing, compared to only 31 per cent of those aged 65 or over and 37 per cent of non-taxpayers. When asked specifically about income tax, the same pattern emerges. The mean amount offered per month in extra income tax paid is £13.46, but this conceals some important variations.

Percentage willing to pay more	All	Non-taxpayers	Basic rate	Higher rate
Higher income tax rate	19	16	22	18
A tax used only for the NHS	44	45	43	47
A charge for visiting the doctor	14	13	14	23
A charge for visiting hospital	6	6	5	2
A higher prescription charge	13	14	13	12
DK	7	9	6	3

The opinions of actual taxpayers indicate some willingness to pay a moderate amount more. The most popular two options chosen were £10 and £11–20, which were in the middle of the list of options given to respondents and therefore the 'middling' option. It is unclear how taxpayers would respond in practice to additional charges of this sort.

What does emerge clearly is public opinion about the priorities for this notional new money which individuals say they would be willing to pay. There is clear support for its being spent on cancer screening (78 per cent for) and new treatments (71 per cent) and clear opposition to its going on so-called 'lifestyle' treatments like tattoo removal (91 per cent against), cosmetic surgery (83 per cent) and infertility treatment (71 per cent).

There is a consistent majority, of approximately two to one, in favour of higher taxation rather than direct charging, although there is a clear preference for a hypothecated health tax over paying into the general pool of income tax.

Comparison with other countries

Level of concern at better treatment in other European countries (per cent)	
Greatly concerned	27
Somewhat concerned	38
A little concerned	21
Not at all concerned	14

The idea that better treatment is available in other countries is obviously disquieting to the majority of British public opinion. Nearly two thirds of the public are concerned about better treatments being available in continental Europe but not in the UK and, surprisingly, as many as 45 per cent would be willing to travel to another country for better treatment if the costs were met by the NHS.

However, when asked for an explanation for differences in the treatments available in Britain and other European countries, there was no consensus answer: 27 per cent did not know; 26 per cent thought it was just that other countries rationed health care in a different way; 22 per cent thought that it was because other countries spent more money on health; 17 per cent thought that the NHS was worse run than other health systems, and 13 per cent that other countries' patients were better informed about their treatments. The answers suggest that willingness to go abroad for treatment or to see other countries' health systems as preferable to the NHS may be largely based on public perceptions that 'the grass is greener on the other side' rather than any substantive knowledge about improved health care treatment and outcomes.

Conclusion

This survey underscores that the public, although generally deferential and satisfied with the NHS, has considerable concerns that they will be negatively affected in the future. People are still generally deferential in their attitudes to health care. Rationing features prominently amongst the public's worries.

Not only is the UK public becoming steadily more aware of rationing as a current concept, and as a future trend (67 per cent expect rationing either to remain at current levels or worsen over the next decade), it is becoming steadily more subtle in its approach. Initial concern is twofold: the length of waiting time for treatment – the most obvious and widely publicised form of rationing – but also the lack of choice in therapies and treatments.

People rely on a range of sources for their health information. Apart from their GP, they consult family and friends, TV and radio and the press. Few use the Internet, and only 20 per cent expect it to become more important as a source over the next decade, although its exponential growth as a source of health information was not predictable even five years ago in the United States.

More information about diseases, and better drugs and technologies are available than ever before. Yet, undoubtedly, the *range* of treatments available from the NHS is becoming gradually more restricted. The survey indicates that there is an emerging conflict between the desire for a greater range of choice and problems arising from the rationing made inevitable by the NHS' funding mechanism. Something will have to give.

The public wants, as the Labour Party detected in opposition, more money to be spent on reducing waiting lists. But it also wants money spent on having the latest and most effective medical technologies and therapies available. The general public is wary that its main concerns will not be addressed without a specifically designated allocation. This leads to considerable support for a hypothecated tax and a significant minority approving of direct funding of the NHS through user charges.

Attitudes and priorities change when one talks about the overall NHS budget and public spending, and individual contributions to the NHS. Asked where their own money should go, the public expressed a preference for it being spent on practical and core services. This includes better consultations with GPs, a wider choice of treatments and medicines, and a reliable appointments system.

If charges are inevitable, as many of the public believe, they want a modern, improved service in exchange. It is the task of government to reconcile these demands with the mixed feelings voters have about how to pay for them.

Appendix

Methodology

In total, 2,048 interviews were conducted face-to-face, in home, among adults aged 18 or over. The research was conducted between 16 and 25 July 1998 at 102 sampling points, based on parliamentary constituencies, throughout the UK. Quotas were set on gender, age, housing tenure and working status. The resulting data have been set to the known population profile.

Profile of respondents

Gender

Female	52%
Male	48%

Age

18–24	11%
25–44	39%
45–64	30%
65+	21%

Number of household members

1	19%
2	34%
3–4	36%

Number of children in household

None	60%
1	15%
2	13%
3	5%
4	1%

Age of children

Aged 0–4	34%
Aged 5–6	25%
Aged 7–8	24%
Aged 9–10	20%
Aged 11–12	22%
Aged 13–14	17%
Aged 15–16	16%

Employment status

Full time	43%
Part time	11%
Not working	46%

Respondent tax status

Basic rate	51%
Higher rate	6%
Non-taxpayer	40%

Partner tax status

Basic rate	39%
Higher rate	4%
No tax	24%
N/A – single person household	22%

Respondents work in a variety of occupations, and of those working in the health service 2% work for the fire, police or ambulance services and 2% are doctors, nurses or hospital workers.

Political Allegiance

Conservative	20%
Labour	43%
Liberal Democrat	10%
None	9%
Refused	8%

Sampling Points

Aberdeen Central
Aberdeenshire West & Kincardine
Aidrie & Shotts
Aldridge Brownhills
Banbury
Batley & Spen
Beckenham
Bedford
Bedfordshire North East
Birmingham Hallgreen
Birmingham Ladywood
Birmingham Perry Bar
Blackpool North and Fleetwood
Blyth Valley
Bolsover
Bolton Northeast
Bradford North
Bradford South
Bristol North West
Broxtowe
Bury South
Camberwell & Peckham

Cambridge
Cambridgeshire Northwest
Cardiff Central
Cardiff West
Carlisle
Carmarthen East & Dinefwr
Carshalton & Wallington
Charnwood
Cheltenham
Chichester
City of London–Westminster South
Colchester
Colne Valley
Congelton
Cotswold
Croydon Central
Cunninghame South
Dartford
Devon East
Dorset West
Dover
Ealing-Acton & Shepherds Bush
East Ham
Edinburgh-Pentlands
Ellesmere Port
Erith & Thamesmead
Essex North
Exeter
Feltham & Heston
Fife Northeast

Glasgow Govan

Grantham & Stamford

Greenock & Invercylde

Greenwich & Woolwich

Guildford

Hampshire North East

Hampshire North West

Hartlepool

Hereford

Heywood and Middleton

Knowsley North and Sefton East

Knowsley South

Leeds Central

Leeds East

Leicester South

Leyton and Wanstead

Lincoln

Liverpool – Riverside

Loughborough

Maidstone & The Weald

Manchester-Gorton

Mid Lothian

Middlesbrough

Mitcham & Morden

Newcastle under Lyme

Norfolk Northwest

Northavon

Oxford West & Abingdon

Putney

Ribble Valley

Richmond (Yorks)
Romford
Saffron Walden
Sheffield Brightside
Sheffield Central
Slough
St Ives
Stockport
Stoke on Trent
Stratford-upon-Avon
Suffolk Central & Ipswich North
Sunderland South
Swansea East
Thanet North
Thanet South
The Wrekin
Tonbridge & Malling
Tyne Bridge
Vale of Clwyd
Walsall North
Warwickshire North
Weston-super-Mare
Wirral West
Wokingham
Worsley
Worthing East & Shoreham
Worthing West
Yorkshire East

NHS opinion survey

Survey questions

Good morning/afternoon. I am from ICM Research, the independent social research organisation. We are conducting a survey in this area and I would be grateful if you could help by answering a few questions. This survey should take about 15–20 minutes. We are interviewing a random selection of people on issues about the National Health Service.

Firstly I would like to record some information about yourself which will help us classify your responses. These answers are totally confidential.

S1.   Sex
Female   52%
Male   48%

S2.   Age: record exact age
18–24   11%
25–34   21%
35–44   18%
45–54   17%
55–64   13%
65+   21%

S3.   Marital Status
Married   55%
Living together 10%
Single   16%
Widowed   11%
Divorced   6%
Separated   1%

S4. How many people live in your household?
Include respondent and any children

I	19%
2	34%
3	18%
4	18%
5	6%
6	1%
7	1%

S5. How many children live in your household (under 16)?

None	60%
I	15%
2	13%
3	5%
4	1%

S6. How old are your children?

Age 0–4	34%
5–6	25%
7–8	24%
9–10	20%
11–12	22%
13–14	17%
15–16	16%

S7. Employment status of respondent

Working full time (30 hrs/week +)	43%
Working part time (8-29 hrs/week)	11%
Not working (under 8 hrs/week)	8%
Housewife	9%
Retired	19%
Unemployed (registered)	4%
Unemployed (not registered but looking for work)	1%
Student	3%
Other (inc. disabled)	2%

S8. What is the occupation of the head of the household?

(listed)

S9. Showcard S9: Which of these applies to you personally?

Pay basic rate income tax only	51%
Pay higher rate income tax	6%
Do not pay income tax	
(either do not work or earn below the allowance)	40%
Don't know/refused	3%

S10. Showcard S9: And which of these applies to your husband/wife/partner?

Pay basic rate income tax only	39%
Pay higher rate income tax	4%
Do not pay income tax	
(either do not work or earn below the allowance)	24%
Don't know/refused	11%
N/A – single person household	22%

S11. Residential status: Is your home …?

Bought with a mortgage	50%
Owned outright by yourself/member of household	21%
Rented from Local Authority	18%
Rented from private landlord	10%
Other	1%

S12. Generally speaking do you see yourself as Conservative, Labour, Liberal Democrat or something else?

Conservative	20%
Labour	43%
Liberal Democrat	10%
Scottish/Welsh National	1%
Green	1%
Other	1%
Don't know	7%
None	9%
Refused	8%

Experience of the NHS

1 Which of the following have you visited in the last year? Showcard 1
2 Ask for each one mentioned: How many times have you visited them in the last year? Read scale

	VISITED	NUMBER OF TIMES VISITED			
		once	2 to 5 times	more than 5 times	don't know
NHS Doctor	66%	23%	49%	24%	4%
Accident and Emergency Dept	15%	72%	20%	1%	6%
Hospital Service (non-Emergency)	22%	46%	39%	10%	6%
Dentist (on the NHS)	40%	43%	49%	2%	6%
None	27%				

3 Ask for each one mentioned: Thinking of your last visit to…how satisfied were you with the quality of treatment provided? Read scale

	SATISFACTION				
	very satisfied	satisfied	not satisfied	very unsatisfied	don't know
NHS Doctor	47%	46%	5%	2%	★
Accident and Emergency Dept.	35%	43%	12%	6%	4%
Hospital Service (non-Emergency)	43%	43%	9%	3%	3%
Dentist (on the NHS)	44%	51%	3%	1%	1%

4 How important do you think ... (Insert from list below)
is in ensuring the NHS provides a satisfactory quality of
service? Read scale

	Very important	Quite important	Not very important	Not at all important	Don't know
The Patient's Charter	46%	33%	7%	2%	12%
Staff commitment	74%	23%	1%	★	1%
Increasing the NHS budget	76%	20%	2%	★	2%
Modern buildings	32%	38%	21%	7%	2%
A local Community Health Council "watchdog"	40%	38%	10%	2%	9%
Being treated as a customer not just a patient	48%	28%	11%	8%	6%

Choices in treatment

5 When you visit your doctor with an illness, how fully
does your doctor discuss what is wrong with you and
how your illness should be treated?

Fully	45%
Briefly	30%
Hardly at all	11%
Never	2%
N/A – not been to doctor	12%

6   If you think of more questions about your illness once
    you've seen the doctor what would you do?

Try to make another appointment	38%
Telephone	24%
Look elsewhere for the answer	9%
Leave questions unanswered	18%
N/A – not been to doctor	12%

7   Many conditions can be treated in more than one way.
    How often does your GP give you *any* choice of
    treatments?

Always	10%
Sometimes	27%
Rarely	17%
Never	33%
N/A – not been to doctor	12%

if never OR N/A, skip to Question 10

8   Showcard 8: When you have been given a choice, of
    these reasons, why do you think this is?

I am being prescribed the latest and most effective treatment available	33%
I am being prescribed a treatment adequate for me to get back to living a normal life	56%
I am being prescribed an inferior treatment because the NHS is short of money	10%
Don't know/not stated	2%

9 When you have been given a choice, how fully have the options been explained to you?

Fully	47%
Briefly	42%
Hardly at all	9%
Don't know/not stated	2%

10 Showcard 10: If you were to ask your doctor to prescribe a specific course of treatment of these, what do you think he or she would do?

Prescribe it to me unless there were good clinical grounds not to do so	35%
Offer me something else but explain the reasons why	25%
Prescribe me what they were going to prescribe me anyway	38%
Don't know/not stated	2%

11 Showcard 11: When you are given a prescription by your doctor, is any of the following explained to you?

	Yes	No	Don't know
The name of the drug	57%	42%	1%
Its ingredients	26%	73%	1%
What it is supposed to do	76%	23%	1%
If it has any potential side effects	68%	31%	1%

12 For medicines to work it is often important to finish the full course of treatment even after you have begun to feel better (this is especially true of antibiotics). When your doctor prescribes a treatment like this how often does he/she tell you to finish it? Read scale

Always	68%
Usually	22%
Sometimes	6%
Occasionally	2%
Never	2%
Don't know/not stated	1%

13 How often do you follow that advice? Read scale

Always	69%
Usually	20%
Sometimes	8%
Occasionally	1%
Never	1%
Don't know/not stated	1%

Service quality at the doctors surgery

14 Showcard 14: Charging already exists for some NHS services such as eye tests, prescriptions and dentistry. If the NHS introduced a £10 charge for visiting your family doctor's surgery what would you expect in return... Read from below?

	Yes	No	Don't know
Better waiting rooms in the surgery	49%	49%	2%
To be seen at the appointed time	89%	11%	1%
To get a fast/immediate appointment	91%	9%	1%
To be given more time by the doctor	81%	18%	1%
To be visited by the doctor	71%	28%	2%
To be seen by a doctor even if you could be attended by a nurse	43%	55%	2%
To be given more information about your illness and more choice in how it was treated	85%	14%	1%
To have more operations conducted at the GP's surgery rather than in hospital	51%	47%	2%

15 If you had a minor illness such as a heavy cold or flu and a visit to the doctor's cost £10, do you think you would you go to the doctor, or not? Encourage respondent to choose a response

Go to doctor	14%
Not go to doctor	85%
Don't know/not stated	★

16 Thinking about the people you know, what do you think
   they would do? Encourage respondent to choose a response

Go to doctor   14%
Not go to doctor   85%
Don't know/not stated   1%

17 If you had a condition that you felt your doctor might
   refer you to a hospital for, and a visit to the doctor's cost
   £10, would you go straight to the hospital or to the
   doctor? Encourage respondent to choose a response

Go to the hospital   65%
Go to the doctor first   34%
Don't know/not stated   1%

18 Thinking about the people you know, what do you think
   they would do? Encourage respondent to choose a response

Go to the hospital   67%
Go to the doctor first   31%
Don't know/not stated   2%

19 Showcard 19: If the money raised by charging for a visit
   to the doctors could go on one of these things which
   one would you like it to go to most?

To your doctor to spend on his/her patients   21%
To cut hospital waiting lists   44%
To prevent some treatments being rationed   22%
To pay doctors and nurses more   9%
To improve facilities for patients in hospital
(individual rooms, better food etc)   8%
Don't know/not stated   1%

Personal knowledge about health

20 How would you rate your knowledge of personal health
  issues? Read scale

Very knowledgeable	10%
Reasonably knowledgeable	40%
Some knowledge	29%
Little knowledge	15%
No knowledge	6%
Don't know/not stated	★

21 How has your knowledge improved over the last
  5 years? Read scale

Greatly improved	13%
Improved a little	36%
No change	47%
A little worse	2%
A great deal worse	1%
Don't know/not stated	★

22 Showcard 22: Where do you get your information of
  personal health issues from?

TV & Radio	41%
Magazines and Newspapers	45%
Internet	3%
Reference books/CD ROMS	13%
Pharmacists	22%
Friends and Relatives	34%
Friends and Relatives in the Health Service	13%
Your GP	44%
Telephone Advice Lines	2%

Information Kiosks			1%
Official Literature and Advertising			15%
Don't have information/no sources			15%

[if don't have information/no sources skip to q 24]

23 Showcard 22: Over the next 10 years which of these
    sources of information do you think you will use more,
    less or about the same?

	More	Less	About the same	Don't know/ Not stated
TV & Radio	26%	4%	64%	7%
Magazines and Newspapers	24%	5%	63%	7%
Internet	20%	8%	54%	18%
Reference books/ CD ROMS	20%	7%	59%	14%
Pharmacists	28%	5%	57%	11%
Friends and Relatives	16%	6%	67%	11%
Friends and Relatives in the Health Service	11%	6%	67%	16%
Your GP	31%	4%	58%	6%
Telephone Advice Lines	10%	9%	65%	17%
Information Kiosks	7%	8%	68%	17%
Official Literature and Advertising	18%	6%	62%	14%

Rationing & co-payment

24 Showcard 24: Because of limits on NHS funding some
   treatments are rationed. That means they are not freely
   available to everyone or else they have long waiting lists.
   Which of these do you think the NHS rations?

	Yes	No	Don't know
Infertility Treatment	76%	19%	5%
Cancer screening	41%	55%	4%
Dentistry	49%	46%	5%
Heart operations for the elderly	62%	34%	4%
Tattoo removals	79%	16%	5%
The latest and most effective drugs and treatments	67%	29%	4%
Cosmetic surgery	80%	16%	4%

25 With new scientific breakthroughs leading to the
   discovery of new treatments do you expect the problem
   of rationing to get better or worse over the next ten
   years? Read scale

Get a lot better	6%
Get a little better	27%
Stay the same	27%
Get a little worse	24%
Get a lot worse	16%
Don't know/not stated	1%

26 What do you expect to happen to NHS waiting lists over
the next 10 years? Read scale

Get a lot shorter	5%
Get a little shorter	25%
Stay the same	26%
Get a little longer	25%
Get a lot longer	18%
Don't know/not stated	1%

27 If new treatments are rationed on the grounds of cost
and older, less effective treatments are prescribed
because they are cheaper, how concerned are you that
rationing will affect you? Read scale

Very concerned	33%
Concerned	38%
A little concerned	21%
Not at all concerned	7%
Don't know/not stated	1%

28 In other European countries some new and better
treatments are more widely available than under the
NHS. To what extent does this concern you? Read scale

Greatly	27%
Somewhat	38%
A little	21%
Not at all	14%
Don't know/not stated	★

29 If the NHS were to meet the cost of new and better
   treatments in other countries for UK citizens, how
   willing would you be to travel to these countries?

Very willing   17%
Fairly willing   27%
Not very willing   26%
Unwilling   29%
Don't know/not stated   ★

30 Showcard 30: Which of the following do you think best
   explains the differences between treatments available in
   Britain and Europe?

The NHS is badly run compared with other
  health services   17%
Other countries spend more money on their
  health services than we spend on the NHS   22%
Patients abroad have more information about
  different treatments and a greater say in how
  they are treated than we do here   13%
Every country rations treatment, they just do
  so differently   26%
Don't know   27%

31 If more money for the NHS would make new and better
   treatments more widely available, how willing would
   you be to personally pay for them (either via direct
   charges or in income tax)?

Very willing   8%
Fairly willing   41%
Not very willing   23%

Unwilling   27%
Don't know/not stated   ★

32 How much more in income tax would you be willing
    to pay per month? Write in using leading zeros eg 0150
    = £150
(listed)

33 Showcard 33: Which of these treatments would you be
    willing to pay more money to the NHS for?

	Yes	*No*	*Don't know*
Infertility treatment	26%	71%	3%
Cancer Screening	78%	21%	1%
Dentistry	38%	60%	3%
Heart operations for the elderly	61%	37%	2%
Tattoo removals	6%	91%	3%
The latest and most effective			
drugs and treatments	71%	27%	2%
Cosmetic surgery	14%	83%	3%

34 If you personally had to pay more for the NHS how
    would you most like to do so? Read scale

Higher income tax rate   19%
A tax used only for the NHS   44%
A charge for visiting the doctor   14%
A charge for visiting hospital   6%
A higher prescription charge for drugs and
   medicines   13%
Don't know/not stated   7%

Thank respondent and close code below: from quota sheet
Area:

North West	11%
North	6%
North East	9%
East Midlands	7%
East Anglia	4%
South East	19%
London	12%
South West	9%
Wales	5%
West Midlands	9%
Scotland	9%

Technical note

The survey was conducted by ICM Research, on behalf of
the Social Market Foundation. 2,048 interviews were conducted, according to a quota, face to face at home in 102
sampling points based on parliamentary constituencies. Per-
centages in tables are from a base of all respondents.

Publications

SMF Papers

1. *The Social Market Economy*
   Robert Skidelsky
   1989   £3.50

2. *Responses to Robert Skidelsky on the*
   Social Market Economy
   Sarah Benton, Kurt Biedenkopf,
   Frank Field, Danny Finkelstein,
   Francis Hawkings, Graham
   Mather
   1989   £3.50

3. *Europe Without Currency Barriers*
   Samuel Brittan, Michael Artis
   1989   £5.00

4. *Greening the White Paper: A Strategy*
   for NHS Reform
   Gwyn Bevan, Marshall Marinker
   1989   £5.00

5. *Education and the Labour Market:*
   An English Disaster
   Adrian Wooldridge
   1990   £5.00

6. *Crisis in Eastern Europe: Roots and*
   Prospects
   Robin Okey
   1990   £4.00

7. *Fighting Fiscal Privilege: Towards a*
   Fiscal Constitution
   Deepak Lal
   1990   £4.00

8. *Eastern Europe in Transition*
   Clive Crook, Daniel Franklin
   1990   £5.00

9. *The Open Network and its Enemies:*
   Towards a Contestable
   Telecommunications Market
   Danny Finkelstein, Craig Arnall
   1990   £5.00

10. *A Restatement of Economic*
    Liberalism
    Samuel Brittan
    1990   £5.00

11. *Standards in Schools: Assessment,*
    Accountability and the Purposes of
    Education
    John Marks
    1991   £6.00

12. *Deeper Share Ownership*
    Matthew Gaved, Anthony
    Goodman
    1992   £6.00

13. *Fighting Leviathan: Building Social*
    Markets that Work
    Howard Davies
    1992   £6.00

14. *The Age of Entitlement*
    David Willetts
    1993   £6.00

15. *Schools and the State*
    Evan Davis
    1993   £6.00

16. *Public Sector Pay: In Search of*
    Sanity
    Ron Beadle
    1993   £8.00

38. *The State of the Future*
Robert Skidelsky, Walter Eltis,
Evan Davis, Norman Gemmell,
Meghnad Desai
1998 £10.00

39. *Reflections on Welfare Reform*
Frank Field
1998 £10.00

40. *The Purpose of Politics*
Oliver Letwin
1999 £8.00

41. *A Cue for Change*
Oliver Morgan
1999 £12.00

42. *The Social Market and the State*
edited by Alastair Kilmarnock
1999 £12.99

Reports

1. *Environment, Economics and Development after the 'Earth Summit'*
Andrew Cooper
1992 £3.00

2. *Another Great Depression? Historical Lessons for the 1990s*
Robert Skidelsky, Liam Halligan
1993 £5.00

3. *Exiting the Underclass: Policy towards America's Urban Poor*
Andrew Cooper,
Catherine Moylan
1993 £5.00

4. *Britain's Borrowing Problem*
Bill Robinson
1993 £5.00

Occasional Papers

1. *Deregulation*
David Willetts
1993 £3.00

2. *'There is No Such Thing as Society'*
Samuel Brittan
1993 £3.00

3. *The Opportunities for Private Funding in the NHS*
David Willetts
1993 £3.00

4. *A Social Market for Training*
Howard Davies
1993 £3.00

5. *Beyond Unemployment*
Robert Skidelsky, Liam Halligan
1993 £6.00

6. *Brighter Schools*
Michael Fallon
1993 £6.00

7. *Understanding 'Shock Therapy'*
Jeffrey Sachs
1994 £8.00

Other Papers

Memoranda/Discussion Papers

21. *Better Government by Design: Improving the Effectiveness of Public Purchasing*
Katharine Raymond, Marc Shaw
1996 £8.00

22. *A Memo to Modernisers III*
Evan Davis, John Kay, Alex de Mont, Stephen Pollard, Brian Pomeroy, Katharine Raymond
1996 £8.00

23. *The Citizen's Charter Five Years On*
Roderick Nye
1996 £8.00

24. *Standards of English and Maths in Primary Schools for 1995*
John Marks
1997 £10.00

25. *Standards of Reading, Spelling and Maths for 7-year-olds in Primary Schools for 1995*
John Marks
1997 £10.00

26. *An Expensive Lunch: The Political Economy of Britain's New Monetary Framework*
Robert Chote
1997 £10.00

27. *A Memo to Martin Taylor*
David Willetts
1997 £10.00

28. *Why Fundholding Should Stay*
David Colin-Thomé
1997 £10.00

29. *Lessons from Wisconsin's Welfare Reform*
J. Jean Rogers
1997 £5.00

30. *The Sex Change State*
Melanie Phillips
1997 £8.00

31. *Freedom and the Family*
William Hague
1998 £5.00

32. *Practical Road Pricing*
Stephen Glaister
1998 £5.00

33. *Education Action Zones: The Conditions of Success*
Robert Skidelsky and Katharine Raymond
1998 £8.00

34. *New Dynamics in Public Health Policy*
Nick Bosanquet and Tony Hockley
1998 £5.00

35. *An Anatomy of Failure: Standards in English Schools for 1997*
John Marks
1998 £10.00

36. *Beyond the PSBR: Auditing the New Public Finances*
Evan Davis and Brian Pomeroy
1998 £8.00

37. *Wanted: A New Consumer Affairs Strategy*
Mark Boléat
1999 £10.00

38. *A Fruitless Marriage? Same-sex Couples and Partnership Rights*
Evan Davis and Melanie Phillips
1999 £5.00

Trident Trust/
SMF Contributions to Policy

1. *Welfare to Work: The* America
   Works *Experience*
   Roderick Nye (Introduction by
   John Spiers)
   1996   £10.00

2. *Job Insecurity vs Labour Market
   Flexibility*
   David Smith (Introduction by
   John Spiers)
   1997   £10.00

3. *How Effective is Work Experience?*
   Greg Clark and
   Katharine Raymond (Foreword
   by
   Colin Cooke-Priest)
   1997   £8.00

Hard Data

1. *The Rowntree Inquiry and 'Trickle
   Down'*
   Andrew Cooper, Roderick Nye
   1995   £5.00

2. *Costing the Public Policy Agenda: A
   week of the* Today *Programme*
   Andrew Cooper
   1995   £5.00

3. *Universal Nursery Education and
   Playgroups*
   Andrew Cooper, Roderick Nye
   1995   £5.00

4. *Social Security Costs of the Social
   Chapter*
   Andrew Cooper, Marc Shaw
   1995   £5.00

5. *What Price a Life?*
   Andrew Cooper, Roderick Nye
   1995   £5.00

Centre for Post-Collectivist Studies

1. *Russia's Stormy Path to Reform*
   Robert Skidelsky (ed.)
   1995   £20.00

2. *Macroeconomic Stabilisation in
   Russia: Lessons of Reforms,
   1992–1995*
   Robert Skidelsky, Liam Halligan
   1996   £10.00

3. *The End of Order*
Francis Fukuyama
1997   £9.50

4. *From Socialism to Capitalism: What is meant by the 'Change of System'?*
János Kornai
1998   £8.00

5. *The Politics of Economic Reform*
Robert Skidelsky (ed.)
1998   £12.00

6. *The Rise and Fall of the Swedish Model*
Mauricio Rojas
1998   £10.00

7. *Capital Regulation: For and Against*
Robert Skidelsky, Nigel Lawson, John Flemming, Meghnad Desai, Paul Davidson
1999   £10.00

8. *Russia: the 1998 Crisis and Beyond*
Kalin Nikolov
1999   £5.00

Stockholm Network

1. *Millennium Doom*
Mauricio Rojas
1999   £10.00

Briefings

1. *A Guide to Russia's Parliamentary Elections*
Liam Halligan,
Boris Mozdoukhov
1995   £10.00

SMF/Profile Books

1. *Is Conservatism Dead?*
John Gray and David Willetts
1997   £8.99

2. *A Better State of Health*
John Willman
1998   £8.99

3. *Will Europe Work?*
David Smith
1999   £8.99